THYROID TRIUMPH

Comprehensive Therapies For Optimal Thyroid Function

Uncover Strategies To Support Thyroid Health And Overcome Common Thyroid Disorders For A Balanced And Energized Life

DR. BRIDGET PROMISE

Table of Contents

CHAPTER ONE

Introduction

Thyroid health is critical for general well-being, yet it is sometimes disregarded until imbalances cause visible symptoms. The thyroid gland, a tiny butterfly-shaped organ located in the neck, is responsible for regulating many biological activities.

In this examination, we will dig into the complexities of thyroid health, including the critical function of the thyroid gland, common problems that might occur, and diagnostic procedures used to diagnose and treat thyroid issues.

Understanding Thyroid Health.

The thyroid gland, a component of the endocrine system, produces hormones that control metabolism, energy levels, and other body activities. The thyroid produces two basic hormones: thyroxine (T4) and triiodothyronine (T3).

These hormones play an important role in managing the body's metabolism, influencing activities including heart rate, temperature, and the rate at which food is converted into energy.

The control of thyroid hormones requires a precise balance. When this equilibrium is upset, it may cause a variety of health problems. An underactive thyroid (hypothyroidism) develops when the gland does not generate enough hormones, resulting in symptoms including weariness, weight gain, and cold sensitivity.

An overactive thyroid (hyperthyroidism) is characterized by an overabundance of thyroid hormones, resulting in symptoms such as weight loss, high heart rate, and anxiety.

The Function Of The Thyroid Gland

To understand the influence of thyroid health on the body, one must first understand how the thyroid gland works. The thyroid gland, located at the base of the neck right under the Adam's apple, secretes hormones into the circulation. These hormones affect the metabolic rate of almost every cell in the body.

When the body requires additional thyroid hormones, TSH stimulates the thyroid to manufacture and release T4 and T3. These hormones are released into the circulation and influence the metabolism of cells and tissues. The thyroid's function in maintaining an equilibrium of energy production and consumption is critical to general health.

Common Thyroid Disorders

Several thyroid problems may alter the delicate balance of thyroid hormone production, resulting in serious health concerns. Among the most common conditions are hypothyroidism and hyperthyroidism.

Hypothyroidism: This disorder arises when the thyroid gland does not create enough hormones to fulfill the body's requirements. Common reasons include autoimmune illnesses such as Hashimoto's thyroiditis, in which the immune system assaults the thyroid, as well as iodine insufficiency. Symptoms of hypothyroidism include tiredness, weight gain, cold sensitivity, and dry skin.

Hyperthyroidism, on the other hand, is caused by an overactive thyroid gland that produces too many thyroid hormones. Graves' disease, an autoimmune illness, is one of the most prevalent causes of hyperthyroidism. Symptoms include weight loss, fast heart rate, anxiety, and heightened heat sensitivity.

Thyroid nodules are another common thyroid condition. These are abnormal growths on the thyroid gland that are often discovered during standard physical exams or imaging examinations. While most thyroid nodules are benign, some may be malignant and need more study and treatment.

Diagnostic Approaches To Thyroid Conditions

Thyroid diseases must be diagnosed using a multidisciplinary approach that includes clinical examination, laboratory testing, and imaging investigations. The first stage is usually a detailed review of the patient's medical history as well as a physical examination. Doctors may ask about symptoms, family history, and risk factors for thyroid disease.

Laboratory testing is critical in evaluating thyroid function. The most frequent blood tests are:

1. Thyroid Stimulating Hormone (TSH): High levels indicate an underactive thyroid, while low

levels indicate an overactive thyroid.

2. Free T4 and Free T3: These tests assess the quantities of unbound thyroid hormones in the blood, giving information on the gland's activity.

3. Thyroid Antibody Tests: These tests aid in the diagnosis of autoimmune conditions such as Hashimoto's thyroiditis and Graves' disease.

In addition to blood testing, imaging techniques like ultrasonography may be used to examine the thyroid gland and detect any abnormalities, such as nodules or inflammation.

In certain circumstances, a radioactive iodine uptake test or thyroid scan may be indicated. These tests entail administering a tiny quantity of radioactive iodine, which allows healthcare experts to evaluate the thyroid's functionality and structure.

Fine-needle aspiration biopsy is a diagnostic method used to detect thyroid nodules. This process involves extracting a tiny sample of tissue from the nodule using a fine needle. The sample is then analyzed under a microscope to see if the nodule is benign or malignant.

Understanding thyroid health is critical for sustaining general well-being since the thyroid gland regulates metabolic processes throughout the body. Common thyroid diseases, including hypothyroidism and hyperthyroidism, may have a significant impact on a person's health and quality of life.

Healthcare practitioners may successfully diagnose and treat thyroid disorders by using comprehensive diagnostic procedures that include clinical examination, laboratory testing, and imaging investigations. As new research sheds light on the complexity of thyroid health, a thorough knowledge of the gland's function and diseases becomes more important for both healthcare practitioners and patients.

The thyroid, a tiny butterfly-shaped gland in the neck, regulates several body activities, including metabolism, energy generation, and temperature regulation. When the thyroid is not working properly, it may result in a variety of illnesses, including hypothyroidism and hyperthyroidism. Traditional therapies for thyroid diseases generally include drugs and, in some situations, surgery. However, holistic viewpoints, dietary techniques, lifestyle treatments, and stress management all play important roles in thyroid health.

CHAPTER TWO

Conventional Treatments For Thyroid Disorders

Conventional therapies for thyroid problems are often condition-specific. Synthetic thyroid hormones, such as levothyroxine, are widely used for hypothyroidism, which occurs when the thyroid gland produces inadequate hormones. This drug helps to normalize hormone levels, which relieves symptoms such as weariness, weight gain, and cold sensitivity.

Hyperthyroidism, or an overactive thyroid, may be treated with hormone-limiting drugs such as methimazole or propylthiouracil. In certain circumstances, radioactive iodine treatment or surgical thyroid gland removal (thyroidectomy) may be indicated.

While these traditional techniques are successful in treating thyroid diseases, they are mainly concerned with symptom relief and hormone level regulation. However, holistic approaches to thyroid health focus on treating the underlying problems and fostering general well-being.

Holistic Perspectives On Thyroid Health

Holistic approaches to thyroid health take into account the interconnectivity of the body, to balance not just thyroid function but total health. These viewpoints often include alternative treatments such as acupuncture, yoga, and meditation, which have been demonstrated to improve thyroid function.

Acupuncture is an ancient Chinese treatment that involves inserting small needles into particular places on the body to enhance energy flow. Some research shows that acupuncture might assist in regulating thyroid function and alleviate symptoms associated with thyroid diseases.

Yoga, which focuses on breath control, meditation, and moderate movement, has been shown to aid people with thyroid issues. Certain yoga positions are thought to stimulate the thyroid gland and promote its normal function.

Meditation and stress-reduction practices are essential for comprehensive thyroid treatment. Chronic stress may impair thyroid function by altering hormone production and the body's delicate equilibrium. Mindfulness activities may help reduce stress, creating a healthy environment in which the thyroid can operate efficiently.

Nutritional Strategies For Thyroid Optimization

Nutrition is essential for maintaining thyroid function. Certain nutrients are required for the production of thyroid hormones, and shortages may lead to thyroid dysfunction. Iodine, selenium, zinc, and vitamin D are some of the important minerals that influence thyroid function.

Iodine, a necessary component of thyroid hormones, is received from the diet, mostly from iodized salt, shellfish, and dairy products. Selenium, present in Brazil nuts, salmon, and sunflower seeds, is essential for thyroid hormone conversion and thyroid protection against oxidative stress.

Zinc, found in meat, nuts, and seeds, helps the immune system and contributes to thyroid hormone synthesis. Adequate vitamin D levels, gained from sunlight and certain meals, are also required for thyroid function.

In addition to maintaining adequate consumption of essential nutrients, some people try gluten-free or autoimmune protocol (AIP) diets to manage thyroid issues. These diets are aimed at reducing possible triggers for autoimmune reactions, which may be important in illnesses such as Hashimoto's thyroiditis.

Lifestyle Interventions For Thyroid Support.

Exercise, sleep, and the management of environmental pollutants may all have a substantial influence on thyroid function. Regular physical exercise has been linked to improved thyroid function and metabolism. Aerobic exercise and strength training both improve general health and may help those with thyroid issues.

Adequate sleep is critical for hormone control and general wellness. Poor sleep quality and inadequate sleep length have been related to hormonal abnormalities, including thyroid dysfunction. Developing a regular sleep habit and treating sleep disturbances may improve thyroid health.

Another significant part of lifestyle treatments is limiting exposure to environmental contaminants, such as hormone-disrupting compounds present in some plastics and pollution. These pollutants may interfere with hormone synthesis and cause thyroid dysfunction.

CHAPTER THREE

The Effects Of Stress On Thyroid Function

Stress, both physical and mental, may have a significant influence on thyroid function. The adrenal glands control the body's stress response, which influences thyroid hormone synthesis and conversion. Chronic stress may cause abnormalities in the hypothalamic-pituitary-thyroid (HPT) axis, upsetting the complex feedback loop that governs thyroid function.

Cortisol, the principal stress hormone, may block the

conversion of the inactive thyroid hormone (T4) to the active form (T3), resulting in hypothyroid-like symptoms. Furthermore, persistent stress may lead to the development or worsening of autoimmune thyroid diseases such as Graves' disease or Hashimoto's thyroiditis.

Stress management via relaxation methods, mindfulness practices, and lifestyle changes is an essential part of maintaining thyroid function. Stress reduction is a common focus in holistic methods to boost general well-being and thyroid function.

To summarize, although traditional medicines are important in the therapy of thyroid problems, holistic viewpoints, dietary methods, lifestyle interventions, and stress management are all important components of comprehensive thyroid care. Integrating these treatments may provide a more comprehensive and personalized approach to thyroid health, treating not just symptoms but also underlying imbalances and contributing factors. Individuals with thyroid issues may benefit from a mix of conventional and holistic methods to improve their overall well-being.

Herbal Treatments For Thyroid Health

The thyroid, a little butterfly-shaped gland in the neck, regulates metabolism, energy generation, and general health. When the thyroid gland does not operate properly, it may cause a variety of health problems, including tiredness, weight gain or loss, and mood swings. While traditional medicine provides excellent treatments such as thyroid hormone replacement therapy, many people choose herbal medicines and alternative therapies to maintain thyroid health. In this investigation, we look at herbal medicines, alternative therapies like acupuncture, exercise routines, mind-body connections via meditation, and the role of functional medicine in supporting thyroid health.

Herbal Treatments For Thyroid Health

Nature has offered several herbs renowned for their ability to support thyroid function. Ashwagandha (Withania somnifera) is an adaptogenic plant often used in Ayurvedic therapy. Ashwagandha is thought to help regulate thyroid hormones and decrease stress, which is a major contributor to thyroid abnormalities. According to studies, Ashwagandha may improve T4 conversion to the more active T3 hormone, which aids in thyroid management.

Another plant gaining popularity is bladderwrack (Fucus vesiculosus), a species of seaweed high in iodine, a mineral required for thyroid function. Iodine is an essential component of thyroid hormones, and a lack may cause thyroid malfunction.

Bladderwrack supplements may benefit thyroid health by supplying the required iodine.

Furthermore, Holy Basil (Ocimum sanctum), often known as Tulsi, contains adaptogenic qualities that may help the body deal with stress and regulate cortisol levels.

Chronic stress is often associated with thyroid abnormalities, and adding Holy Basil into one's daily routine may help to improve general thyroid health.

CHAPTER FOUR

Exploring Alternative Therapies: Acupuncture And Thyroid Harmony

Acupuncture, an ancient Chinese medical method, involves inserting small needles into particular places on the body to enhance energy flow and balance. In terms of thyroid health, acupuncture is thought to assist control of the endocrine system, which includes the thyroid gland. By focusing on particular acupuncture sites linked to hormonal balance, practitioners hope to restore thyroid equilibrium and enhance general health.

Several studies show that acupuncture may affect thyroid hormones and alleviate symptoms associated with thyroid diseases. While further study is required to properly demonstrate acupuncture's effectiveness, many people have reported excellent results when combined with conventional thyroid therapies.

Thyroid-Friendly Exercise Regimen

Regular exercise is necessary for good health, and it may be especially helpful for those who have thyroid problems. Engaging in thyroid-friendly workouts, such as moderate aerobic activity and strength training, may assist in improving metabolism and weight control, both of which are significant problems for people with thyroid abnormalities.

Yoga, in particular, has gained appeal for its mild yet effective approach to thyroid health. Certain yoga postures, like the shoulder stand (Sarvangasana) and the fish position (Matsyasana), are said to stimulate the thyroid gland and enhance hormonal balance. Yoga's attentive and stress-reducing character may also have a great influence on general well-being, helping to maintain thyroid equilibrium.

Mind-Body Connections: Meditation And Thyroid Harmony

Thyroid health is heavily influenced by the complex relationship between the mind and body. Chronic stress, typically caused by contemporary lifestyles, may contribute to the development or worsening of thyroid diseases. Meditation, a discipline aimed at resting the mind and lowering stress, has emerged as an effective approach for achieving thyroid equilibrium.

Mindfulness meditation, in particular, enables people to be present in the moment, which promotes serenity and reduces the effects of stress on the body. According to studies, daily meditation may alter the release of stress hormones and improve thyroid function. Integrating meditation into your daily practice will benefit not just your thyroid but also your general mental and emotional wellness.

Functional Medicine And Thyroid Wellness

Functional medicine is a holistic approach to healthcare that focuses on identifying and treating underlying causes of health problems. In the context of thyroid health, functional medicine practitioners strive to identify the underlying reasons for thyroid abnormalities, taking into account nutrition, lifestyle, and environmental variables.

Comprehensive testing may be used in functional medicine to check thyroid function, nutritional levels, and probable sources of thyroid problems. Functional medicine seeks to restore overall health and promote thyroid well-being by recognizing and correcting systemic abnormalities.

Finally, herbal medicines, alternative therapies such as acupuncture, thyroid-friendly exercise regimes, meditation, and functional medicine concepts all contribute to a comprehensive approach to thyroid health.

While these techniques should not be used instead of traditional medical treatments, they may be beneficial in increasing general well-being for those with thyroid issues. Individuals contemplating alternative remedies should always speak with a healthcare practitioner to obtain a thorough and tailored thyroid care plan.

Navigating Hormone Balance For Thyroid Health

The thyroid, a tiny butterfly-shaped gland in the neck, regulates a variety of body activities.

Maintaining optimum thyroid health is critical for general well-being because it produces hormones that regulate metabolism, energy levels, and mood. In this thyroid health inquiry, we will look at the complicated web of hormonal balance, the influence of thyroid drugs, empowering self-care methods, real-life success stories, and a road map to optimum thyroid function.

CHAPTER FIVE

Understanding Thyroid Medications And Their Impact

Understanding the function of drugs in thyroid problems is critical for controlling the illness. Thyroid drugs are often administered to manage hormone levels and come in a variety of forms.

The two most frequent forms are liothyronine (T3) and levothyroxine (T4). Levothyroxine is a synthetic variant of the thyroid hormone T4, while liothyronine is a synthetic version of T3. Maintaining healthy thyroid function requires balancing the appropriate dosages of these drugs.

It's crucial to understand that thyroid medicine might take some time to take effect. Regular monitoring of hormone levels via blood tests is required to modify medication doses as necessary.

Age, weight, and metabolism may all have an impact on how well thyroid medicine works. Collaboration with healthcare experts guarantees effective treatment and reduces any negative effects.

Patient Empowerment: Self-Care Techniques For Thyroid Triumph

Empowering individuals to actively engage in their thyroid health is an important element of treating thyroid diseases. While medicine is necessary, self-care techniques may have a substantial impact on overall well-being.

1. Proper Nutrition: A balanced diet rich in iodine, selenium, and zinc promotes thyroid function. Seafood, dairy, almonds, and seeds may all help offer the nutrients you need.

2. Stress Management: Chronic stress may negatively impact thyroid function. Meditation, yoga, and deep breathing techniques may help manage stress and promote hormonal balance.

3. Regular exercise boosts general health and improves thyroid function. Regular exercise, even a daily stroll, helps to improve metabolism and energy levels.

4. Adequate Sleep: Proper sleep is necessary for hormonal balance. Establishing a regular sleep habit and developing a sleep-friendly atmosphere are critical stages in maintaining thyroid health.

5. Make Healthy Lifestyle Choices: Limiting smoking and alcohol intake is excellent for thyroid health. Additionally, being aware of environmental issues, such as toxin exposure, might help to maintain a healthy thyroid.

Success Stories: Personal Journeys To Thyroid Wellness

Knowing that others have overcome similar obstacles and attained thyroid health may be motivating for those on their paths. Success tales often emphasize the tenacity of people who have overcome thyroid diseases via a mix of medical treatment and lifestyle adjustments.

Consider Sarah, who, after years of tiredness and inexplicable weight gain, was diagnosed with hypothyroidism. Sarah undertook pharmaceutical changes and adopted a holistic approach to her health, as advised by her healthcare staff. Sarah restored energy and lost weight by committing to regular exercise, a thyroid-friendly diet, and stress-management skills.

These examples highlight the significance of individualized approaches to thyroid health.

What works for one person may not work for another, highlighting the need for tailored treatment and a thorough knowledge of the variables impacting thyroid function.

Closing Thoughts: Your Roadmap To Optimal Thyroid Function

Managing hormonal balance for thyroid health requires a comprehensive approach. Recognizing the interdependence of lifestyle, medication management, and tailored treatment is critical to promoting normal thyroid function.

As you begin your path to thyroid health, consider the following roadmap:

1.   Educate   yourself. Understanding your thyroid status, medicines, and the influence of lifestyle choices allows you to take an active role in your healthcare journey.

2. Establish a Support System: Surround yourself with helpful healthcare professionals, friends, and family. Having a network that understands and supports your efforts may make a big impact.

3. Prioritize Self-Care: Include self-care techniques in your everyday routine. Prioritize acts that benefit your entire well-being, such as a balanced diet, frequent exercise, or stress-management skills.

4. Regularly evaluate and adjust your thyroid hormone levels using blood testing. Collaborate carefully with your healthcare providers to alter medication doses as appropriate and address any new concerns.

5. Recognize and appreciate milestones in your thyroid health journey. Recognizing your efforts

and accomplishments strengthens your dedication to maximum well-being.

Conclusion

To summarize, the process of achieving hormonal balance for thyroid health is both customized and dynamic. Individuals may achieve higher well-being by understanding thyroid drugs, empowering self-care routines, drawing inspiration from success stories, and following a plan for healthy thyroid function. Individuals who actively manage their thyroid health may live a better, more vibrant life.